Dr. Martha's 52 weeks of victorious Aging

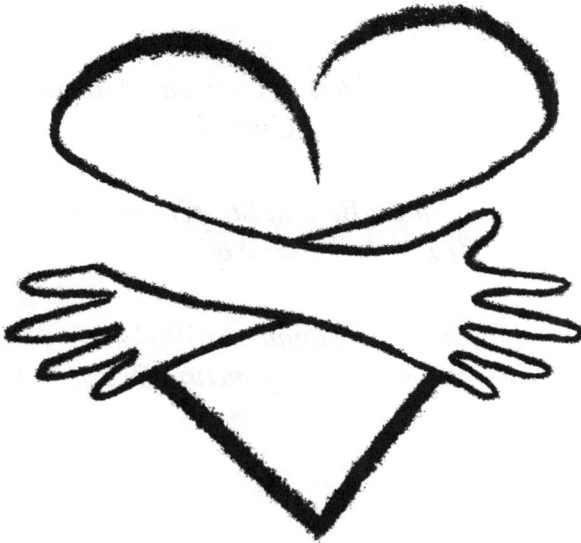

Tips to Ensure a Happy and Healthy Year at Any Age

Also by Dr. Martha Lucas

Catholic Daughters of Catholic Mothers:
A Memoir and Guided Journal

Pulse Diagnosis: Beyond Slippery and Wiry:
Key to the Practice of TCM!

Cosmetic Acupuncture Works!:
Your Guide to Cosmetic Acupuncture for Anti-Aging

Dr. Martha's 52 weeks of victorious Aging

Tips to Ensure a Happy and Healthy Year at Any Age

Dr. Martha Lucas, L.AC.

WWW.ACUPUNCTUREWOMAN.COM

Armlin House Productions

Dr. Martha's 52 Weeks of Victorious Aging: Tips to Ensure a Happy and Healthy Year at Any Age Copyright © 2023 by ArmLin House Productions

Cover Artwork & Illustrations Copyright © 2023 by Wendy Spurlin

ArmLin House Productions
P.O. Box 2522, Littleton, Colorado 80161-2522

ISBN: 978-1-958185-21-6

Cover Design by Wendy Spurlin Designs
www.wendyspurlin.art

Printed in the United States of America

First Edition

Fall in love with taking care of yourself. Fall in love with the path of deep healing. Fall in love with becoming the best version of yourself but with patience, with compassion, and respect to your own journey.

F. S. McNutt

Introduction

I have been practicing Traditional Chinese Medicine for over 20 years, and its basic premise is that we can live long, active, and healthy lives. This lifestyle is achievable by learning about healthy options that, when implemented, can result in an improved physical and emotional well-being.

This book offers active tips that will create a healthier, happier you as you advance in years– what I call Victorious Aging. The actions presented will tap into the healing power of your own body and spirit. What's wonderful is that many of the activities cost nothing to achieve significant results.

Here's what one reader told me:

"I have this book on my Kindle so that I can read a weekly tip and strive to reach that mindset or goal. And I often refer to the tip throughout the week. It's a great little bible of useful information for me."

I've provided 52 health and happiness actions that you can realistically incorporate into your life. I thought long and hard about a 365-day book but, having bought one or two in my day, I realized that 365 is too much pressure. Most of us don't need another thing to do each day, let alone try to remember to read every day. Once a week is perfect. Set an alarm or reminder to start the week with a tip, read an entry midweek, or end your week with your choice of advice.

Also notice that there are no dates in the book. It doesn't start on January 1st like similar health and happiness books do. This is because you can start this practice on any day or week in the year. In fact, your birthday is a great time to commit to improve your health and thrive in your Victorious Aging journey!

Tips to Ensure a Happy and Healthy Year at Any Age

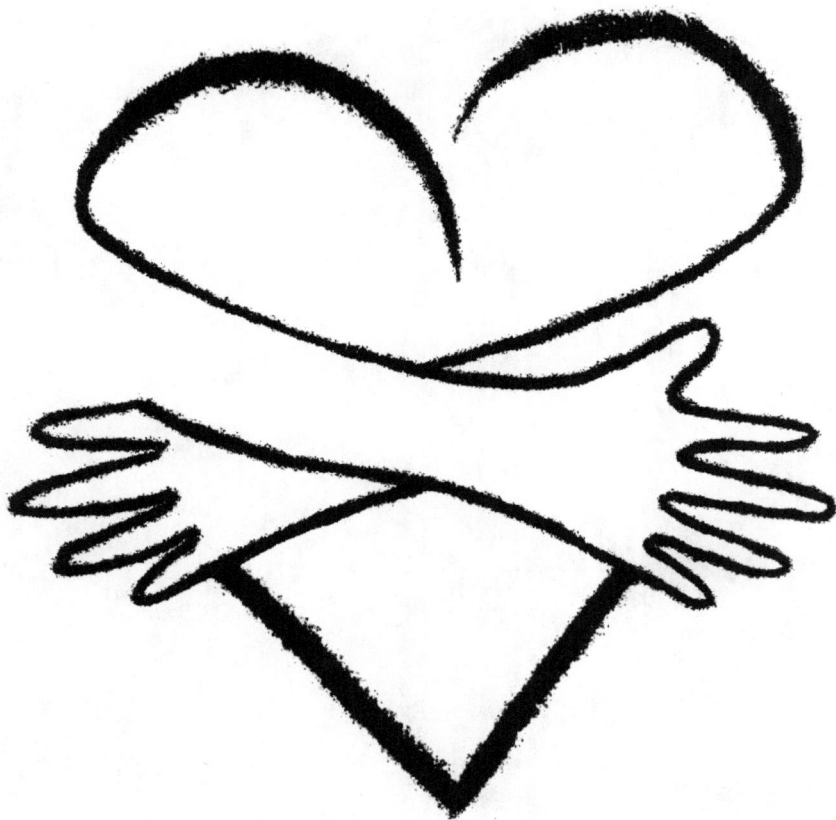

1. Like Yourself

Yes, like yourself.

Or how about this crazy idea—LOVE yourself!

Loving yourself means having regard for your own well-being and happiness.

It means that you act in ways that support your physical, emotional, and spiritual growth.

You take care of your own needs; you know how to say, "no." You don't sacrifice your own well-being.

Focus on what is good within you and maximize your positive qualities.

Basically, develop a good relationship with yourself, and celebrate the beauty and freedom of being you every day!

2. unplug

Unplug: take a screen vacation…

Try it for an hour each day this week to see if you feel refreshed and calmer.

Some years ago, I went on a wagon train adventure where there was no cell service. While I was uncomfortable at the start of the trip that it would include 5 days without phones or other electronics, I remember feeling more relaxed than I had in a long time. Being in constant touch with literally everyone/everything takes energy and attention. The break was good!

Unplugging improves sleep habits, increases creativity, and develops interpersonal communication. It can even make you more productive!

3. smell some sunscreen

Yep, that's right! The smell of sunscreen can make you feel happier. Why? Because it reminds you of relaxing on sunny days at the beach, picnicking in the park, lounging in your backyard, and even vacationing with family when you were a kid.

Its perfume creates an association with more stress-free or relaxing times that elicits a rush of happiness.

Smell is our most primitive sense and one of our most powerful. Of all the senses, it is the most effective trigger of memories. When a particular bouquet is paired with a pleasant memory, happiness is revived when we whiff the same scent in the present. It's not the scent per se, it's the past happy memory associated with the scent that makes us feel good.

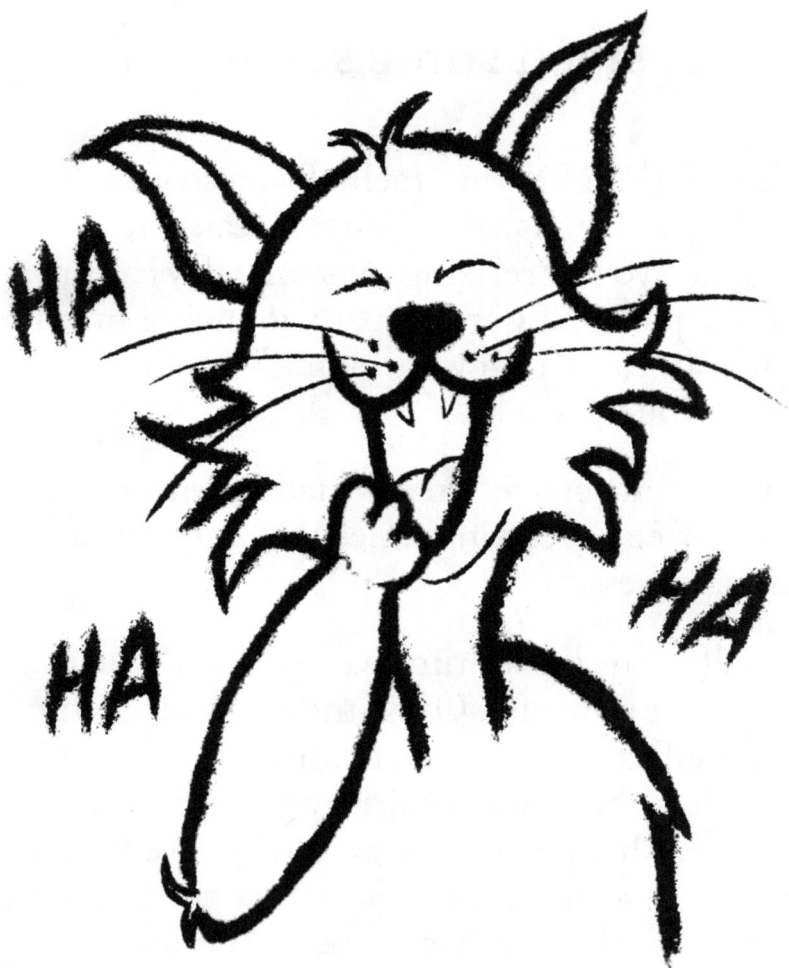

4. Laugh out Loud

If you want to relieve stress, the Mayo Clinic says, "Giggles and guffaws are just what the doctor ordered."

Laughter forces your lungs to take in more oxygen.

It increases endorphins, the feel-good hormones in your brain.

A good laugh relaxes your muscles and helps your body produce its own natural painkillers.

In the long run, laughing makes your immune system work better, lifts your mood, and just plain improves your health.

5. Hug

Get your daily hug.

Yep, daily. At least one hug every day this week!

Hugs heal.

Receiving and giving hugs releases endorphins and other good chemicals that reduce stress. Reducing stress helps us be healthier and happier.

Hugs can lower your blood pressure, boost your immune system, and even reduce depression.

6. Take a walk

Take a walk in the park or around your neighborhood. Greet neighbors.

Hippocrates, the father of medicine, said, "If you are in a bad mood, go for a walk. If you are still in a bad mood, go for another walk."

We've all heard that it's important to move our bodies to stay healthy. Walking is a way to maintain a healthy weight and prevent diseases like heart disease, stroke, high blood pressure, and type 2 diabetes.

So, a walk a day keeps the doctor away!

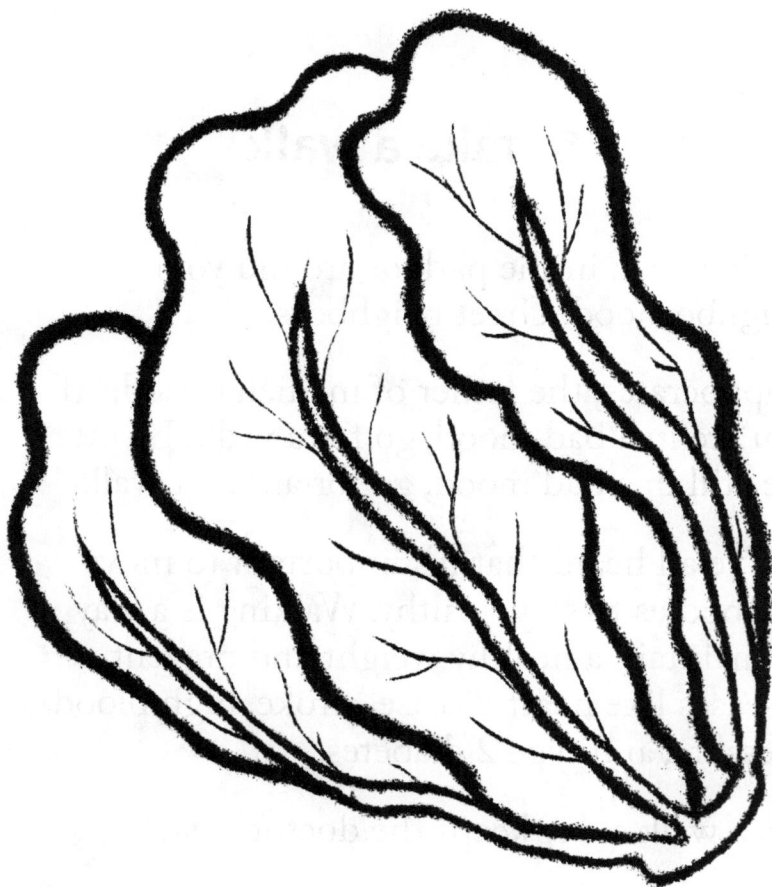

7. Eat Lettuce

Enjoy a big bowl of lettuce.

Researchers in the UK conducted a study they actually named Lettuce Be Happy to highlight the health and mood benefits of eating lettuce.

The leafy vegetable is an excellent source of vitamin K, which helps to strengthen bones.

Eating lettuce helps you get a good night's sleep, keeps your eyes healthy, and hydrates your body—but don't forget water too!

How about trying a few different varieties of lettuce this week?

8. smile in Front of a Mirror

Smile at yourself in front of a mirror.

You can do this every day when you brush your teeth, comb your hair, do your nasal wash…

You get the idea.

Smiling—even if you're just instructed to smile and it's not a genuine or Duchenne smile—influences your physical body.

For example, smiling while we are in a stressful situation, even if it is a fake smile, calms us down.

In other words, the action of forming a smile reduces the intensity of your body's stress response, even if you don't feel happy.

So, the next time you're stuck in traffic, turn up that smile, and you'll be more able to "grin and bear it."

9. Eat Blue Potatoes

Improve your memory and mood by eating blue potatoes.

You can mash them, roast them with some olive oil, or even make homemade low-sodium potato salad. Add onions and celery for some extra zing and crunch.

Blue potatoes get their color from anthocyanins, powerful neuroprotective antioxidants that improve your short-term memory. They also reduce inflammation—the bad boy implicated in so many chronic health conditions.

And blue potato skins supply lots of iodine to regulate your thyroid, which reduces tiredness and depression.

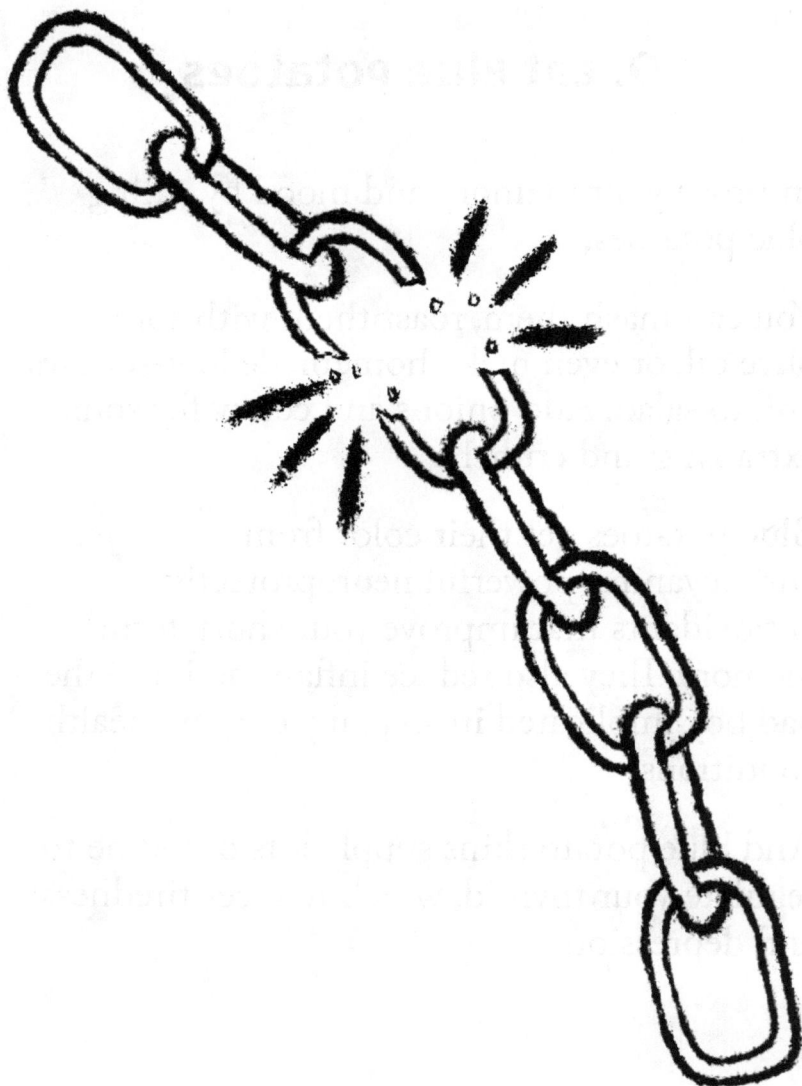

10. Break a Bad Habit

We all form bad habits we'd like to break. Most habits annoy us, but we just can't seem to quit indulging in that cookie before bed!

Our brain loves patterns or routines, aka "habits." They're difficult to break because your brain doesn't want you to stop them.

I often explain this to my patients, whom I see for releasing/resolving trauma patterns. Not only does their brain strengthen the habits, but it also resents that there's some lady (me) who's trying to make it change!

Anyway, it's best to do these things to diminish unhealthy patterns:

- Intend it; intend to break the bad habit.

- Enlist support from family and friends.

- White knuckle it through the behavior change.

- Be ready for successful change that isn't a straight line.

- Celebrate your successes and improved health!

11. Eat some Yogurt

Serotonin is a brain chemical associated with happiness and satisfaction.

Did you know that the gut produces 80% of the body's serotonin? This means that having a healthy digestive system has a direct effect on how happy you feel.

Why yogurt? Because it is a probiotic food. These foods maintain or improve the good flora in your body, reducing inflammation and boosting your immune system.

And it's full of nutrients in and of itself: calcium, B vitamins, magnesium, vitamin D, and protein.

Read the label on the yogurt package so you don't choose one that contains too much sugar.

12. Accept Your Greatness

Spend time with people who recognize your greatness, even if you don't or aren't ready to accept it in yourself.

They are the people you trust, and they are friends you enjoy having a relationship with.

They love and admire you; love them back.

Accepting yourself and being open to compliments is important for healthy relationships, as well as for your good health.

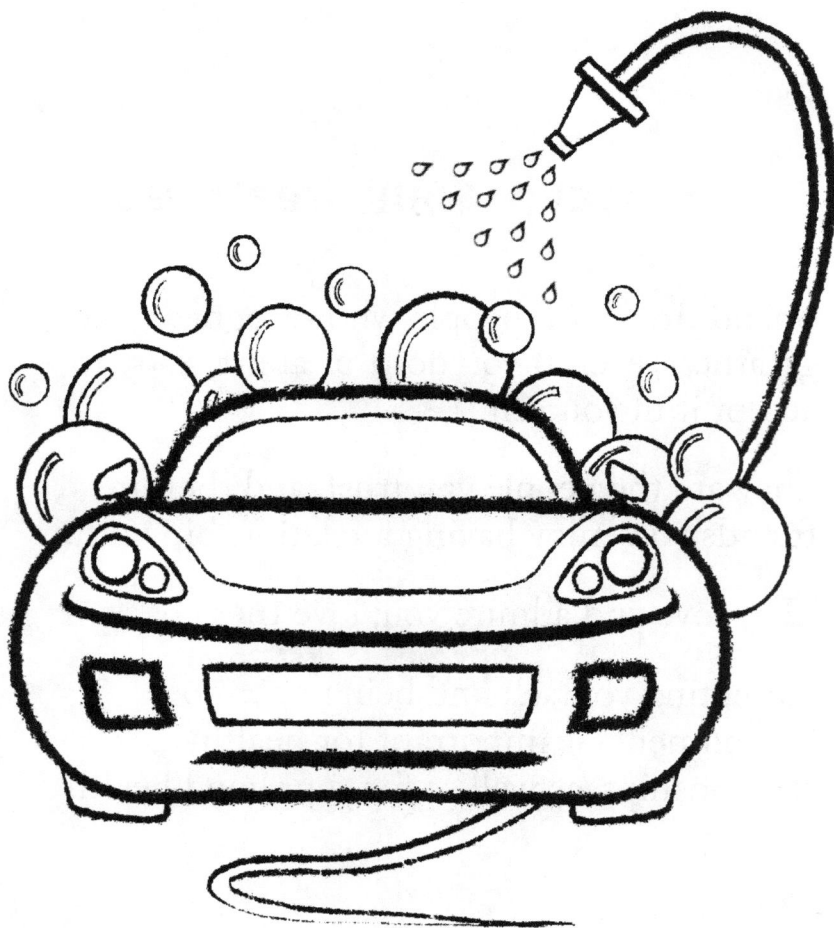

13. Wash Your Car

Gather a bucket, sponge, and hose, and wash your car.

Grab the Windex and get those windows sparkly. Vacuum the mats and floor, then stand back and admire your work!

Turns out that having a clean car makes you feel happy.

And studies have shown that a clean car makes you feel healthier and less stressed, besides feeling overall happier.

14. Pamper Your skin

Take care of your skin.

It's your largest organ and includes functions like regulating body temperature and protecting you from germs.

Wear sunscreen every day.

Moisturize morning and night.

Use a non-drying cleanser.

Use a moisturizing scrub once or twice a week.

And try a mask… it's so easy. Take it out of the jar, put it on your face, neck, and décolleté, then relax and let it work!

15. Lean into Lean Proteins

Lean protein in a 100-gram portion contains less than 10 grams of total fat and fewer than 4.5 grams of saturated fat.

Lean protein supplies your body with the vitamins and minerals that it needs to run efficiently.

It's an excellent source of protein, vitamin B12, zinc, and iron.

Eating lean protein lowers cholesterol, preserves muscle and bone, and supports brain function.

Remember that preserving muscle and bone not only contributes to a healthier life but a longer one.

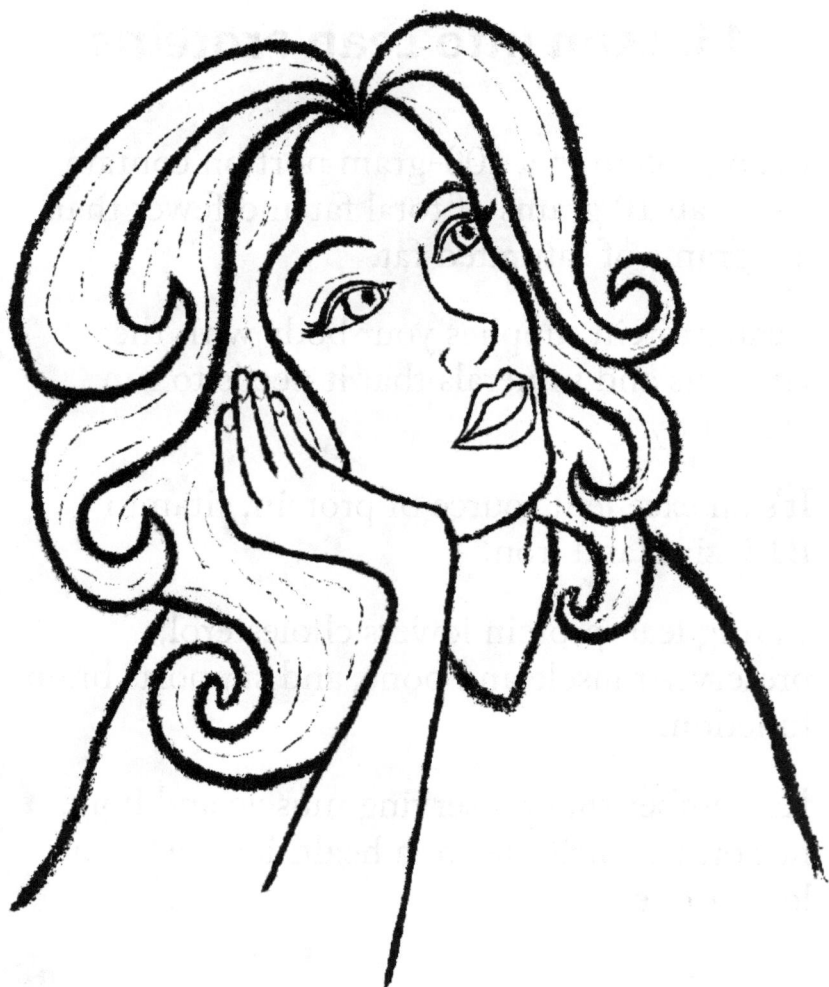

16. Daydream

It's surprising how often your brain is in "daydreaming" mode.

And it's a function of the brain that has significant benefits.

So let your mind wander.

Daydreaming enhances creativity and boosts problem-solving abilities. That's right! Sometimes the wandering mind solves a problem better than thinking about the problem directly.

Daydreaming helps to reduce stress and anxiety, leading to a healthier you.

17. Make a choice

Make a choice, any choice.

The ability to choose things for yourself, or free will, is an essential part of happiness.

It turns out that free will isn't just a philosophical concept. The ability to choose things for ourselves plays a vital role in increased life satisfaction.

Studies show that people with higher free will experience lower stress, higher life satisfaction, more meaningful lives, and greater levels of bliss.

Simply making a choice—what to eat for breakfast, what to do during free time, who to date or marry—is a powerful source of happiness.

So, recognize your power to choose and make a choice!

18. Eat Tomatoes

Eat tomatoes and tomato products.

Tomatoes are a significant source of vitamin C, beta carotene, potassium, folate and other B vitamins, iron, and fiber.

Eating cooked tomatoes in products like pasta sauce allows for the absorption of a very potent antioxidant called lycopene. Lycopene has anti-cancer properties and improves your skin's health.

Tomatoes help protect heart health, prevent constipation, prevent type 2 diabetes, boost your immune system, and support male fertility.

They're exceptionally good for your health!

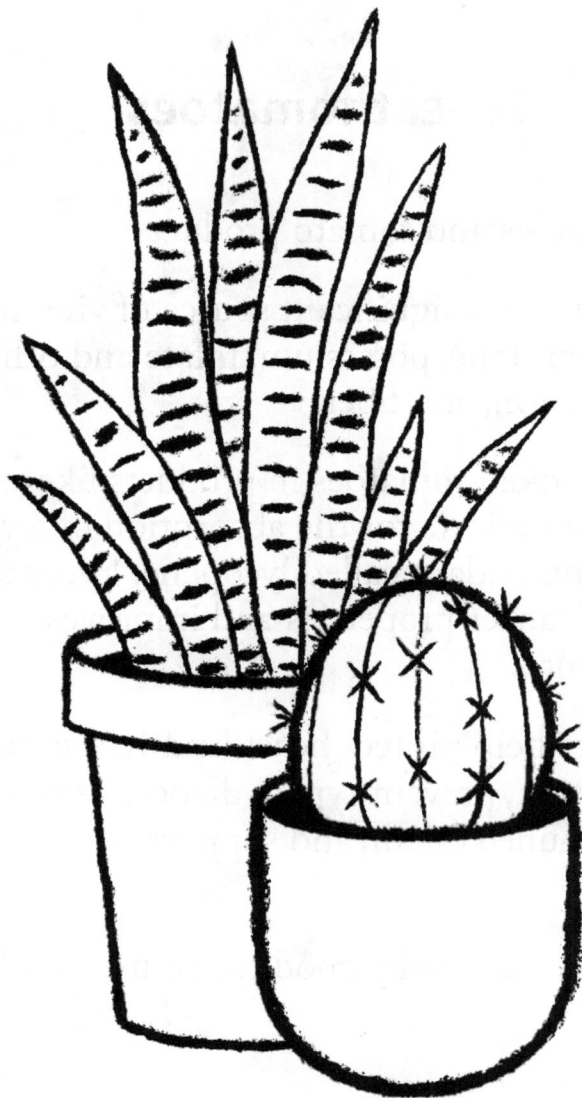

19. Talk to Plants

Talk to your plants. Ask how they are doing.

Believe it or not, plants respond to the vibrations of nearby sound—you talking to them—which activates two important genes for their growth. And they respond better to nice calm speech, not yelling.

We also benefit from hanging out with plants and conversing with them. It gives us a psychological boost, calms us down, and promotes our emotional and physical health.

Don't forget to check up on the amount of sunlight they can absorb, their watering schedule, and their soil content.

Just like you take care of your health, take care of theirs.

20. call an old friend

When's the last time you called an old friend?

You've heard the saying, "The important things in life aren't things."

It's not the things, it's a person or people. Human beings are an ultra-social species. It's our nature, and we can't live without personal interactions.

Relationships with family and friends are crucial to achieve happiness throughout your life.

Heaps of studies have concluded that social connections make people happy.

In fact, some studies suggest relationships are necessary for better health, content feelings, and a longer life.

21. Be Flexible with Food

When eating healthy, flexibility works best. Don't restrict yourself to a certain way of eating or only eating certain types of foods if that type of eating doesn't work for you.

When people come to me for weight loss, we start with my Lighten Up! program. It helps people determine what type of eating schedule they prefer and what type of movement/ exercise suits them.

One of my main points is that the program, the plan, the diet must be enjoyable so that you succeed. If you try to follow an inconvenient plan, you won't comply with it. If you eat unappetizing foods, you won't stick to your diet. If recipes are complicated, you won't prepare the right meals.

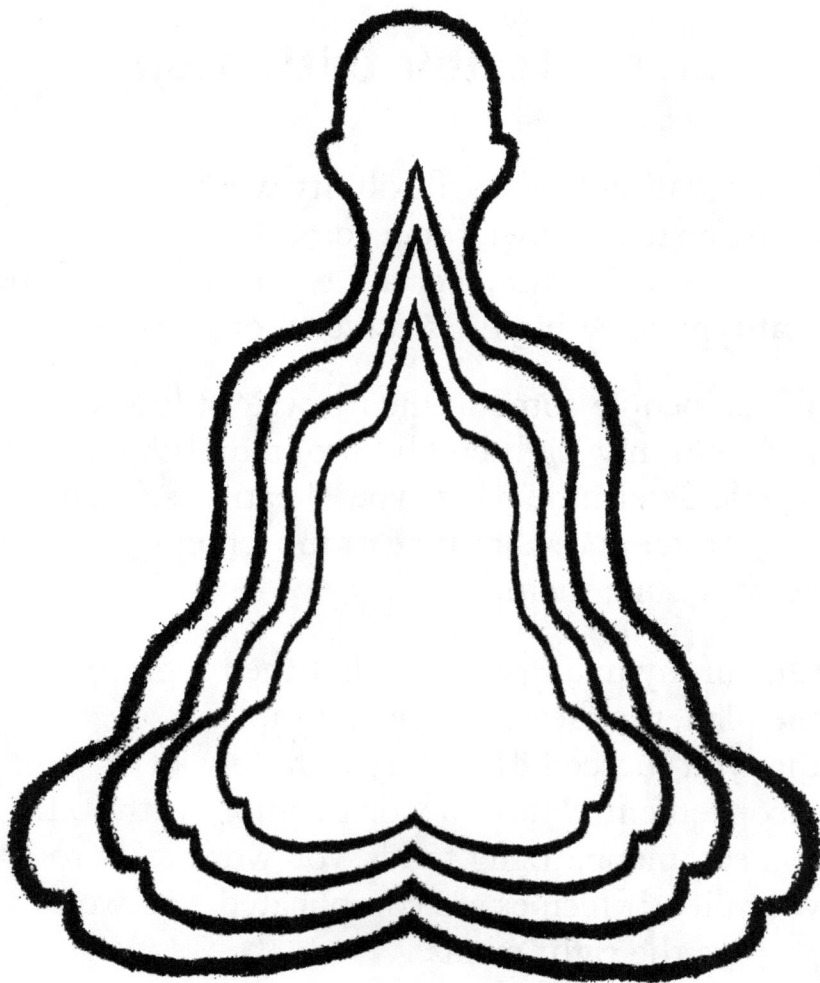

22. Breathe Deeply

Take a deep breath.

For just a few minutes a day, practicing a calming breathing technique will make you feel healthier and happier.

In fact, studies have showen that breathing techniques like Sudarshan Kriya yoga can help alleviate depression.

Deep Belly Breathing 5, 7, 3 is a simple breathing technique that I recommend to my patients. Here's how it works:

1. Breathe deeply into your abdomen for a count of 5.

2. Exhale, pulling your belly in toward your spine for a count of 7.

3. Stop and hold for a count of 3.

4. Repeat 5 more times.

23. Be spontaneous

Try to be spontaneous or do something new each week.

Spontaneity requires a sense of curiosity and openness to step outside of your comfort zone and try new things. Or it encompasses repeating an experience that you just feel like doing today!

When you avoid being spontaneous, you risk getting stuck in a routine, and you may miss out on experiences that bring joy to your life.

Spontaneity opens doors to new perspectives, opportunities for growth, and new relationships.

Plus, you may even experience a new wonder in the world.

- Take an unplanned road trip.

- Stay up late and stargaze.

- Rearrange your furniture.

- Or get up early and watch the sunrise.

24. Print Photos

Photos are little time capsules of a moment. Holding printed photos makes the memories more tangible so you can cherish memories.

There was a time when our photos weren't digital. I remember those days when you couldn't take an unlimited number of photos and hope one would turn out well. Film was in a camera, with a limited number of shots. You tried to make every shot perfect. Then, you'd pay to develop the roll of film. Now, you can literally take 100 shots of a scene, and later, delete 99 of them.

Gather a cute photo of someone you know, put it in a pretty frame, and send it as a gift.

Make a photo album for someone. One Christmas, I gave my grandchildren a photo album containing their baby and adolescent pictures.

Consider these 3 keys to happiness: planning, enjoying, and remembering an event. Preserve this by printing photos of the event.

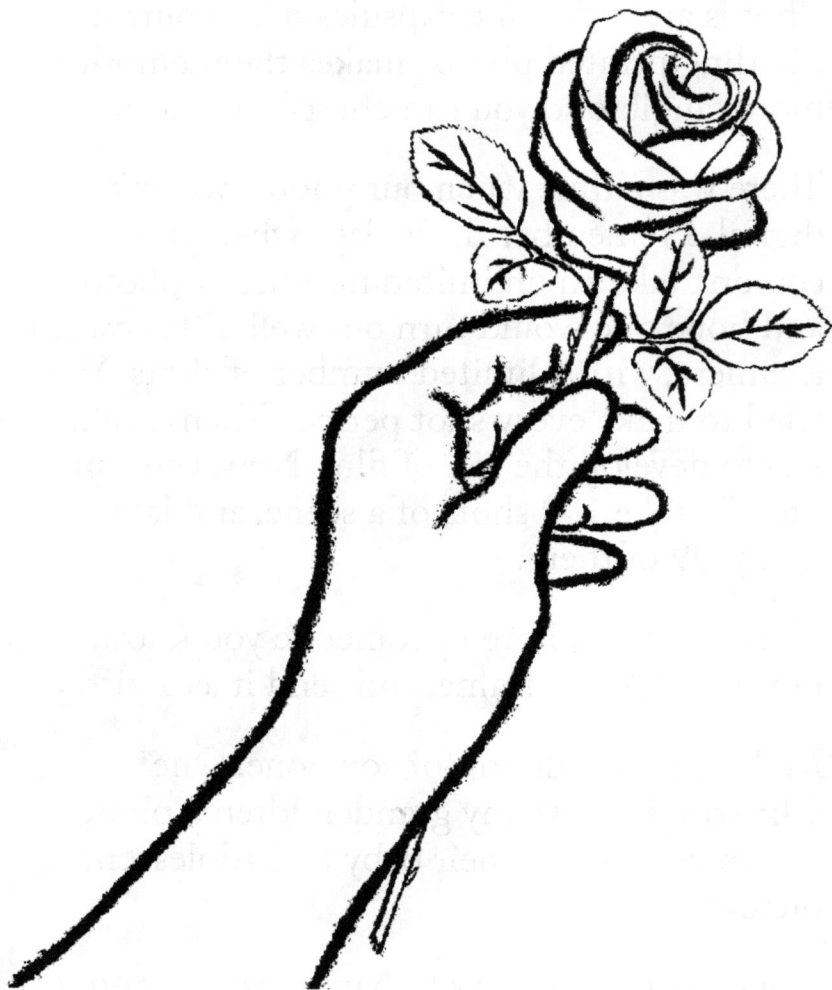

25. Do something Nice

Do something for someone else. It doesn't have to be something big.

Helping someone benefits your physical and mental health. You would think that it just makes you feel good emotionally, but helping others has amazing physical benefits too.

Helping others reduces stress, boosts your immune system, reduces anger, makes you calmer, and reduces pain. And some studies show that helping others can help you live longer.

You've seen bumper stickers or signs that suggest random acts of kindness. Well, research shows that random acts of kindness have a stronger effect on well-being than more formal acts such as volunteering at a shelter.

This week, help someone carry their groceries, leave a positive comment on a blog, listen to a friend. There will be plenty of opportunities to help someone. Even smiling at stranger could improve her day.

26. Express Love

Tell people you love them.

While I don't want to make you sad, years ago, my mother died suddenly. I was very blessed to have spoken with her the night before she died. We had a pleasant conversation and ended our talk by saying, "love you." My brothers, on the other hand, didn't have that opportunity.

I also had a beloved mentor die suddenly, and both deaths taught me that everyone I love needs to know that I love them.

Let people know how important they are to you. People appreciate it; it makes them feel good.

If someone makes you happy, let them know!

There are lots of ways to do it too. You can call. You can meet. You can write a letter that they can keep.

This saying is true: "The most important things in life aren't things."

27. Explore Your Neighborhood

Check out an unexplored part of your neighborhood.

I recently did this myself. I've lived in the Capitol Hill neighborhood of Denver for almost 30 years. I had never visited some streets that were no farther than 8 blocks from my house. One summer evening, I walked these streets. I love looking at houses, noticing their paint colors, observing yard art. And I met new people!

How did I meet them? It was simple. Because it was summertime, people were in their yards, so I stopped to talk with them. I shared that I lived close by but had never been down their street before, then the conversation went from there.

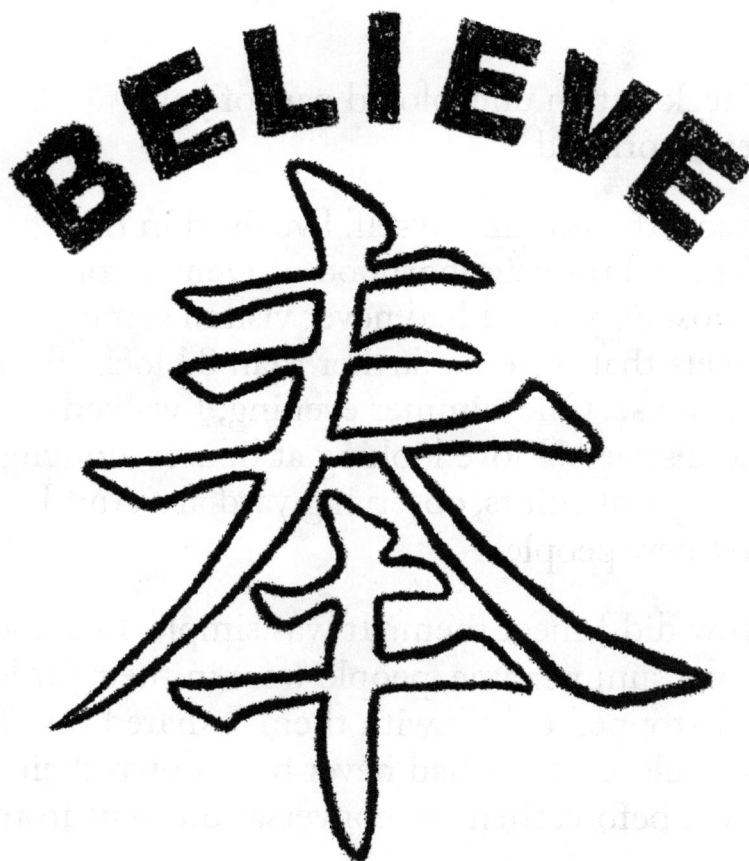

28. Believe in self

Ask yourself, "What do I believe about my life?"

The first time I saw this question, my answer was, "My life is all about sadness and worry and fear." Yes, that was my first answer. Oh boy... That answer made me really think about the question, and I realized, "No, my life is not only about sadness and worry." But why was that my first answer?

It took more time thinking and talking with myself to realize that everyone has moments of sadness and worry, but I don't believe that my life is all about that. Not in the least.

Asking the question and paying attention to the answer allowed me to recognize that sadness and anxiety are only a tiny part of the pie of my everyday life.

So, ask yourself, "What do I believe about my life?"

29. cook with Fresh Herbs

Fresh herbs contain higher concentrations of antioxidants: health-boosting compounds. One tablespoon of oregano and marjoram supplies a ton of antioxidants.

Fresh herbs have more flavor. Their flavor is more potent after they're dried, put into bottles, and left on the shelf.

Herbs help with digestion. Mint, parsley, dill, turmeric, garlic, and ginger all aid digestion.

Chinese medicine has an entire arm about nutritional advice, which includes herbs. For example, ginger has been used for centuries to treat nausea.

30. Learn Your Name in a Different Language

Learning your name in different languages allows you to experience and appreciate different cultures.

Boost your brain power and memory by learning a new language. It keeps your mind sharp.

Some say that learning a new language improves decision making and benefits listening skills and problem solving.

Improving your brain is a lifelong activity.

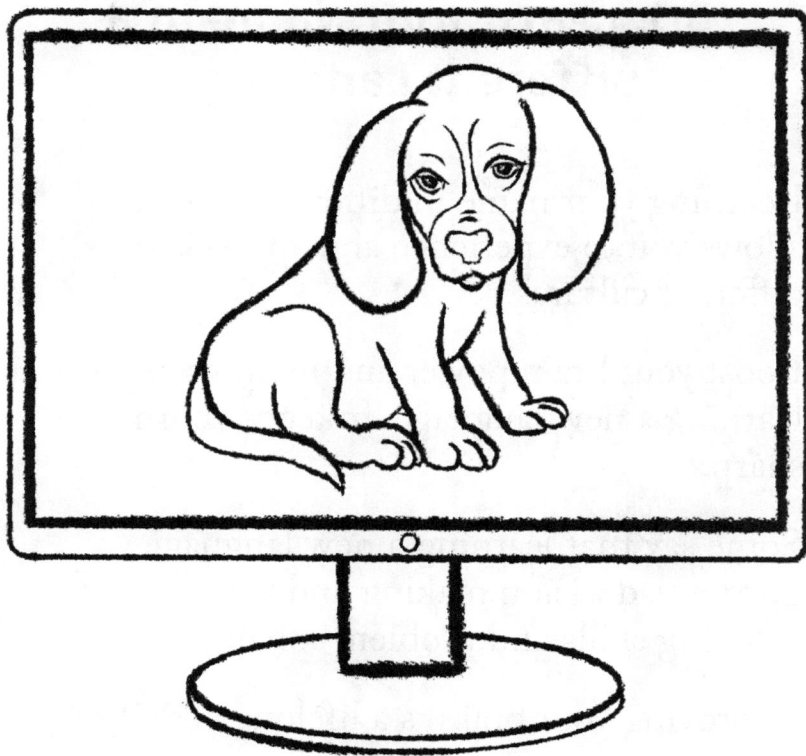

31. change your computer screen

Change your computer screen saver or background to a picture that makes you smile.

We are hard-wired to feel good when we look at something that makes us smile.

It can be a picture of smiling faces.

It can be a quote about happiness.

Sometimes, no matter what we do, we can't seem to hold on to a lasting sense of happiness. That's okay because happiness is not a permanent feeling. It's something that we can define for ourselves, like when we are walking along a trail of fallen leaves while noticing a purple fall flower.

32. Make a Time capsule

Maybe you've only heard of this idea in movies, but making a time capsule preserves moments in time, especially a specific time in your life.

Assemble things representative of a specific time or from the here and now. These items can include newspaper clippings, store catalogs, a menu from your favorite restaurant, or coins. Or write a special note with thoughts of the day. Gather photos and label them with the time that they were taken and add the names of the people in the photos. Seal them in a container, then bury it in your garden, or hide it somewhere in your house, careful to avoid bug or water damage. Dig up the capsule 10 years later.

The entire process will promote joy, boost curiosity, and cultivate wonderful memories—all components of stress relief.

33. Rethink your wardrobe

Try on all your clothes and determine whether they "spark joy" a la Marie Kondo.

If all the clothes in your closet spark joy—think about it—you'll always feel happy when you're in your closet. You'll look good and feel good.

This practice allows you to enjoy what you have and who you are at this moment.

Is there guilt in giving away clothes that don't spark joy? Absolutely not! Even clothes that mean something to you, like an old t-shirt you received as a present but never wore. Be grateful for your relationship with the gift giver, then put the shirt in a box to donate it. Appreciate the love shown by the person who gave you the gift, then let go of the shirt.

Believe me, it won't take much time. You will know right away whether something sparks joy. You'll never worry whether you should keep something, it's too expensive to give away, or you might wear it someday.

Just take a deep breath and spark some joy!

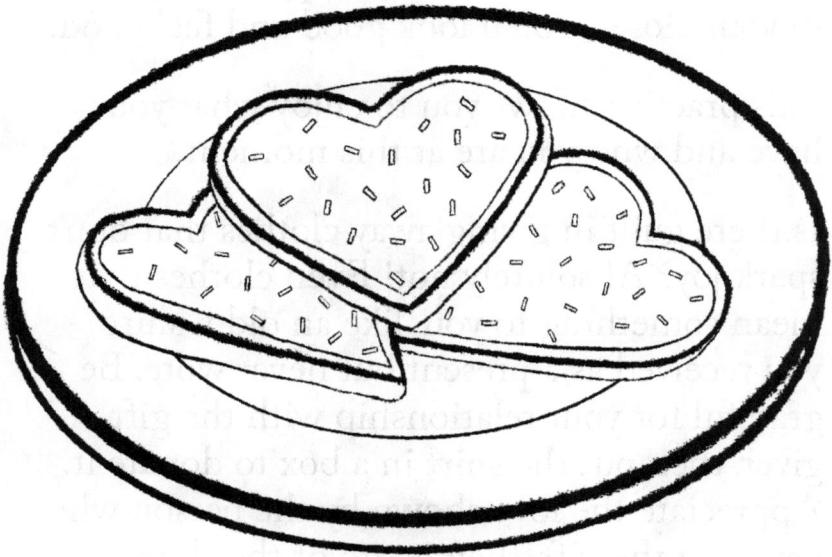

34. Bake Cookies

The smell of baking cookies makes us feel good.

Studies have shown that in malls, when people walk by a store that is pumping out the smell of fresh-baked cookies, they are more likely to help a stranger.

Our sense of smell is our most powerful sense for recalling memories.

Scents are memories ingrained in our minds. They are nostalgic triggers.

A bakery's aroma brings back the pleasant feeling of being in the kitchen with our mother or grandmother during the best of times.

There's a strong connection between scent and emotional well-being, and studies show that it reduces stress and improves mood.

It's about a time when life seemed simple and smelled good.

35. chart Your Emotions

Each day, make a pie chart of your emotions.

Draw a circle on your calendar or just a piece of paper.

Then, when you feel an emotion, make a line or a triangle on the chart to represent how much of the day you felt that emotion.

This is a highly effective visual way to see how much of the day you are happy, anxious, sad, etc.

Guess what? Most days, you will find your pie chart predominantly shows happiness.

36. Experiment in the Kitchen

Some people were born chefs, but there are plenty of us who struggle to whip up meals in the kitchen. The act of cooking, in and of itself, provides time to experiment with different recipes, ingredients, tastes, and skills.

I recently learned how to make a bagel with two ingredients—yes, two! You mix self-rising flour with plain yogurt, knead the dough a bit, and bake. Simple and tasty!

In addition, use this time to try some healthier recipes.

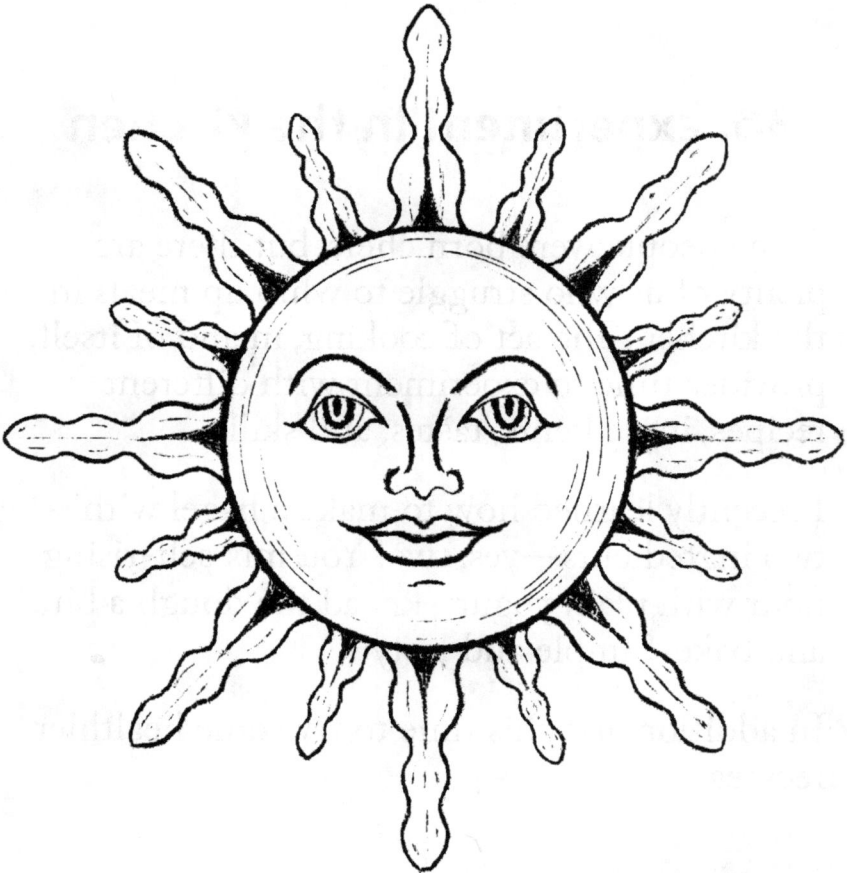

37. Get More vitamin D

I can't say enough about vitamin D. In my practice, I recommend taking 10,000IU a day. During flu season, everyone seems to be sick with some sort of virus. I take 20,000IU a day to help me stay healthy, but check with your doctor for the right dosage for your body.

Vitamin D boosts your immune system, increases muscle mass, and builds strong bones. Wait… isn't that the saying for milk?

You get vitamin D from some foods: fish, dairy, and fortified food products.

The most common source of vitamin D is the sun. Being out in the sunshine for 15 - 30 minutes a few times a week gives you adequate vitamin D. But after 15 minutes, you need sunscreen.

You can ask your doctor for a blood test if you are unsure whether you are getting enough vitamin D.

38. Eat Sweet Potatoes

Eat sweet potatoes. Yum!

Even though they taste sweet, they don't have more calories than white potatoes.

They are root vegetables, high in fiber and antioxidants, that help to promote a healthy gut and brain. And listen to this…a baked sweet potato contains 3 times the recommended daily amount of beta carotene and half the recommended amount of vitamin C.

They are delicious baked, and I like to roast them as French fries too. I just roll them in some olive oil, toss them with a little salt, and roast them in the oven.

39. Use Your Non-Dominant Hand

Attempt to do things with your non-dominant hand: anything from brushing your teeth to using the TV remote to writing a note.

It improves your brain's fitness and stimulates your brain's cognitive and creative fitness.

I take pulses—patients' pulses to determine diagnoses—using my nondominant left hand. For one thing, it allows me to take notes with my right hand. But more importantly, my entire brain is more active and more developed. I believe, and research supports, that I have created more connections between my brain's hemispheres than someone who never uses their nondominant hand.

Your brain adapts and grows new neurons from mental stimulation. Remember the saying, "use it or lose it?" It totally applies to your brain. If you don't use it, it loses knowledge. This is the reason some elderly people have trouble recalling memories (unless the loss of memory resulted from disease.)

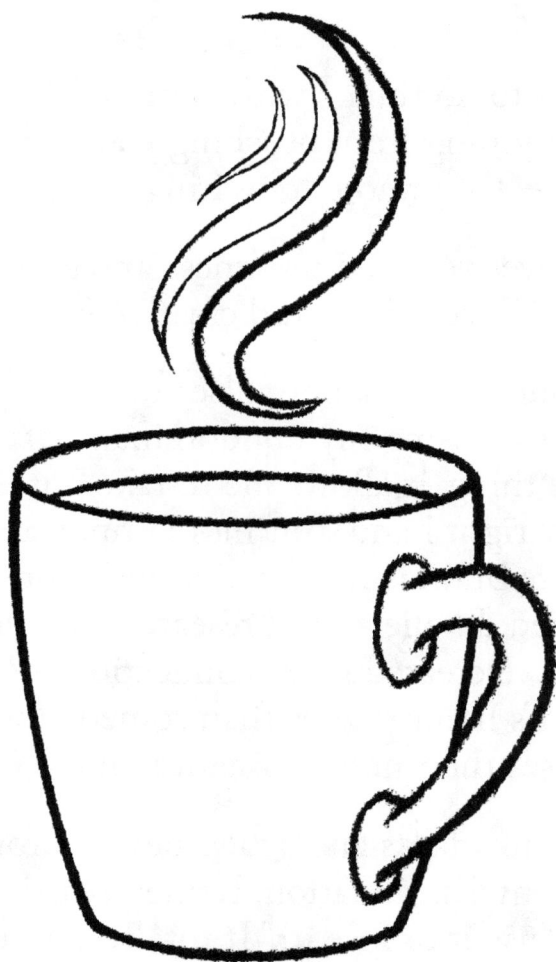

40. Drink coffee

It's okay to drink coffee.

Johns Hopkins Medical Center reminds us that coffee isn't only about caffeine. It is also rich in antioxidants and other substances that may reduce inflammation…the precursor to a lot of diseases.

Turns out that people who drink more coffee are less likely to get type 2 diabetes…so maybe it helps your body process glucose more efficiently. And this one is the most fascinating to me—dark roast coffee can make your DNA stronger; it helps reduce breakage in DNA strands. That's cool because such breakage can lead to disease.

Some research has found that coffee may even reduce your chances of developing Alzheimer's disease, dementia, and heart disease.

So, drink on!

41. Buy Yourself Flowers

You are beautiful, amazing, fabulous…what other reason do you need to spoil yourself occasionally?

Flowers are such a treat for a small cost.

And it's self-care. Remember, self-care is one of the most important things you can do for yourself. Besides pampering yourself, flowers are an instant mood-booster, add color to your home, and fill a room with refreshing fragrance.

Usually, flowers are gifted to moms or loved ones. Why? Because we know a bouquet will make them feel good. We know they will love them. So, why not treat yourself?

42. Be a Mentor

Help someone learn something. You will enable someone else's personal development.

Be a motivator. Mentees stay on track knowing that someone is there to help them reach their goals. Mentors keep mentees accountable.

You will become a trusted ally as you give much needed guidance.

Studies show that both the mentor and her/his pupil experience less anxiety, which improves general well-being.

Teaching others is rewarding and elicits joy and self-confidence.

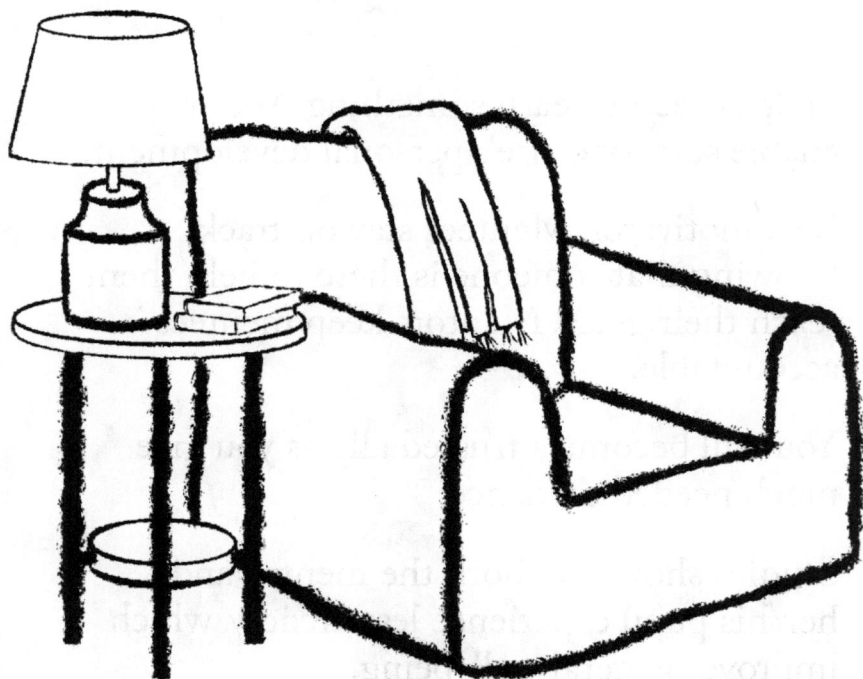

43. create a calm space

Create your own Calm Space to relax. Set aside a place in your home, such as a quiet sitting area with a favorite chair. Make a point of visiting this space daily to unwind and recharge.

Have a natural element present like some greenery.

Declutter—clutter creates anxiety.

Illuminate your calm space with soft and yellowish light—it reduces tension and promotes a feeling of calm.

Involve your senses. Listen to sounds of nature or calming music. Smell essential oils. Touch a super soft blanket or wiggle your toes through a rug under your feet.

Put your electronics away. It's best to take a break from checking emails or notifications.

Display things you love and make the space a reflection of you: your family, your values, your priorities, your story.

Create a space that you love!

44. Forget the Bad Times

Forget about something that made you unhappy. Let go and lead a happy life.

If you can have negative thoughts, you can have positive thoughts. Try to swap out sad or negative thoughts for some positive self-talk.

Work on achieving a growth mindset, which means our skills, thought patterns, and even feelings are developed through practice. It's about improving what you do and how you do it—including your thought process.

It's a lifelong process of learning and awareness so that you can connect to your essence and create happy or calm moments of each day.

45. surprise someone

Deliver a surprise.

Send flowers, baked cookies, or a note to someone.

Guess what? Surprising someone is just as enjoyable for the giver as it is for the receiver. While you are creative in the planning process, there is a buildup of excitement before the act or event.

Surprise works on the dopamine system in our brain, making us feel good physically and emotionally.

Recall past surprises that you have received and how good that made you feel. I still remember being surprised by a note that my Dad left for me in my high school locker. I was trying out for the dance team, and he left a good luck note in my locker. It made both of us feel good!

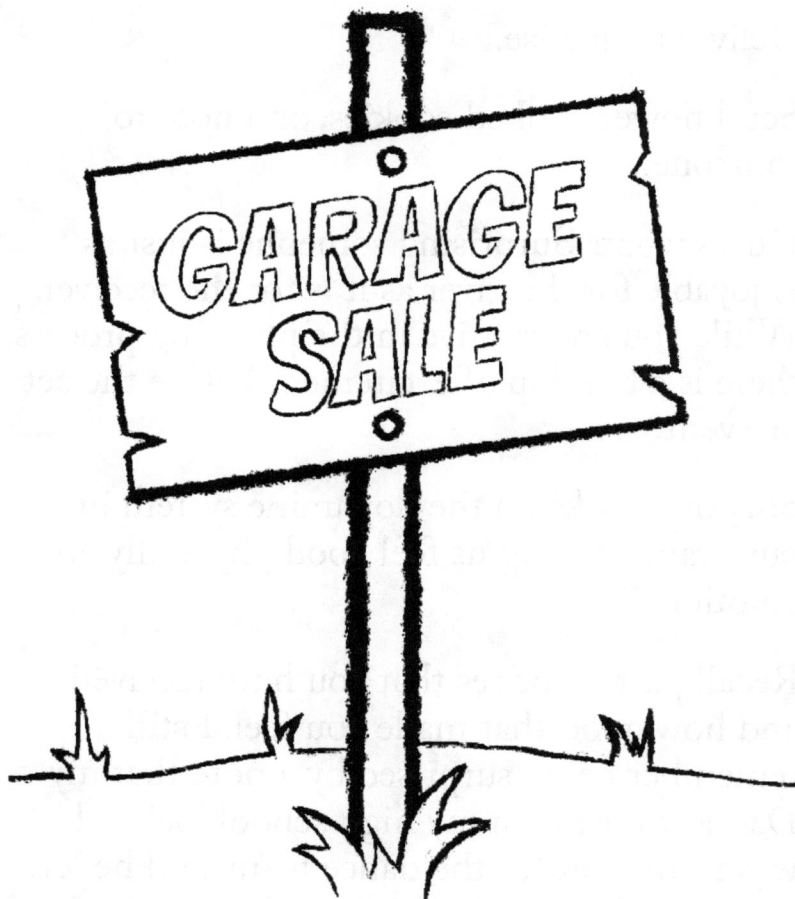

46. Have a Garage Sale

Clear out all your unused clutter, set up a table in your driveway, and have a garage sale. You'll make some cash instead of keeping the stuff in storage or hauling it in to donate.

I often think that I'd be willing to have someone pay me to take the stuff, but it's the other way around. And the buyers are happy; they love your stuff.

It's also a great way to network with your neighbors while refreshing them with cold lemonade or cocktails.

Lastly, you will help the environment by repurposing the items rather than putting them in a dump. Maybe a buyer will sew a quilt with your old clothes or turn your old electronics into a piece of art.

47. watch the sunrise

Get up early to watch the sunrise.

Everyone deserves to start the day with something beautiful, and most people view sunrise and sunset as beautiful events of nature. But watching the sunrise has actual physical benefits:

- Support of your immune system by providing vitamin D

- Balance of your circadian rhythm, which improves your overall body wellness.

- Improvement of your mood by relieving stress and depression.

Watching the sunrise starts your day with positive vibes; you get to start your day on a path of positivity. And think about how peaceful the early morning is. You begin your day in a state of tranquility.

Plus, spending time in nature, or even just observing it, reduces mental fatigue and boosts concentration.

48. Figure out Your Mantra

In ancient Sanskrit, *man* means mind and *tra* means release. I love the idea that a mantra is a mind release. The sound of a mantra releases your mind from the anxieties of material life. The most common mantra is *Om,* but you can establish your own word, group of words, or even hum.

It's a phrase or affirmation that will motivate and inspire you to be your best self, affirm the way you want to live your life, and focus your mind to achieve a goal. It can be a unique expression of what you desire most.

Think of a mantra as a chant. Chanting creates thought-energy waves, and your body vibrates in the energy and spirit of the chant. Chanting a mantra synchronizes the left and right sides of the brain and promotes alpha brain waves. And relaxing mantras improve your health.

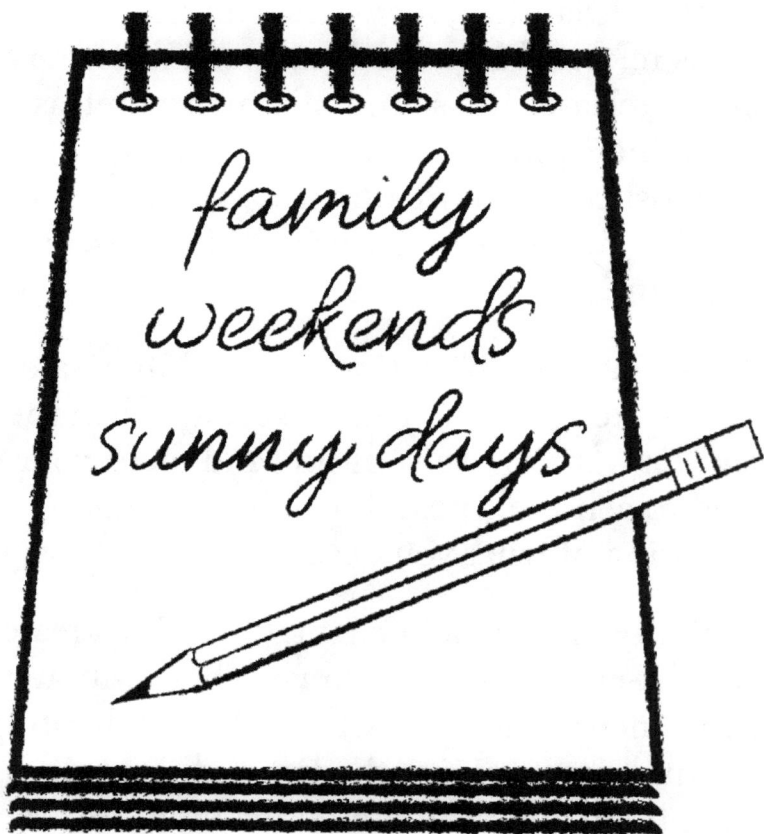

family weekends sunny days

49. start a Gratitude List

Make a list of things for which you are grateful.

This is pretty self-explanatory. You're probably rolling your eyes because you've heard it over and over again. Repetition is how we remember things.

Don't like the idea of a list? Then make a gratitude jar with pretty pieces of colored paper.

Ground yourself and focus on the good in your life. It's things like a cup of coffee, a good night's sleep, flowers on your desk, a loving pet, and the list goes on.

Health-wise? People who practice gratitude sleep better, experience less pain and inflammation, choose healthier options, and are less anxious and depressed.

50. stretch

Work on your flexibility.

Stretching decreases stiffness and injuries. It also enables your muscles to work more effectively and your joints to move through their full range of motion. And your posture will improve.

It both prepares your body for exercise and helps to reduce post-exercise achiness.

Stretching counteracts stress because it activates your parasympathetic nervous system, which triggers a sense of calm and relaxation.

Last but not least, if you stretch before bedtime, it rejuvenates your body while you sleep.

51. Try something New

Try something new. It's good for you!

Whatever new activity you try, promise yourself not to strive for perfection. Focus on engaging your curiosity.

Attempting something new improves memory and mood because it supplies a hit of dopamine, which is one of the feel-good chemicals in our brain.

Plus, the brain continues to develop throughout life, so you might as well train it to do new things.

Pursuing new things also increases adaptability. You overcome fear and resistance when you do something new and outside of your comfort zone.

It's likely, while you are building a healthier brain, you will also acquire new skills and encounter fun, enlightening experiences.

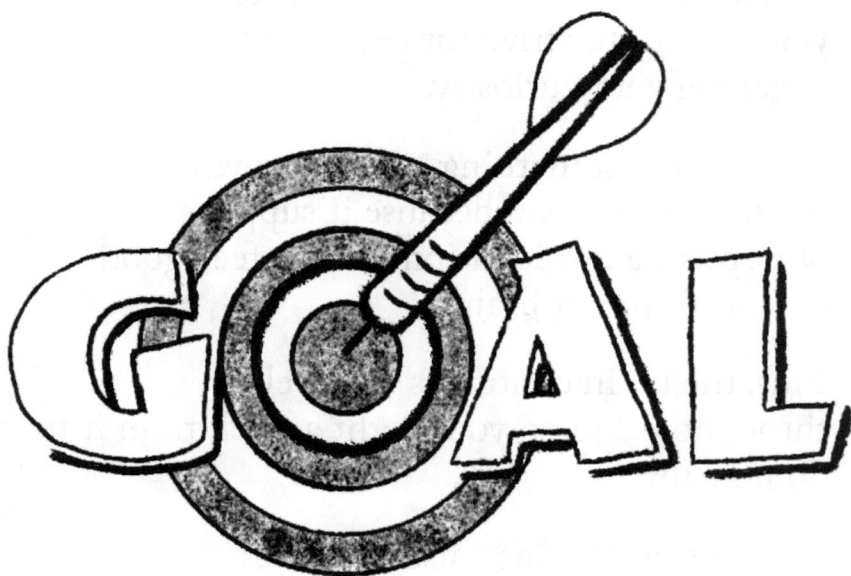

52. Reflect on Accomplishments

Take time to reflect.

What have you accomplished in the last year?

What goals are you setting for yourself in the next year?

Look at the highs and the lows, the wins, and the losses.

Give yourself feedback and look forward to improving each year.

Acknowledgements

I want to thank my mentor, the late Dr. Jim Ramholz, for introducing me to Chinese medicine pulse diagnosis and the power that making a proper diagnosis has in creating effective treatment plans for my patients. Still, after more than 20 years of practicing this medicine, I smile when I feel how acupuncture changes the energetic pattterns in my patients' pulses. It is truly amazing.

And I can't forget my family, friends, and editor, who encourage me while I'm in the middle of my writing projects. Time spent on projects aside, to me, family really is first, and I make time to create new memories with them as well as hope to always have these opportunties.

References

Cormick, G. et al. (2019, July). Calcium intake and health. *Nutrients.*

Dudeja, J.P. (2017, June). Scientific analysis of mantra-based meditation and its beneficial effects: An overview. *International Journal of Technologies in Engineering and Management Sciences.*

Dweck, D. (2007). *Mindset: The new psychology of success.* Random House Publishing Group.

Gordon, S. (2021). The relationship between mental health and cleaning. *Verywell Mind.*

Herz, R. (2016, September). The role of odor-evoked memory in psychological and physiological health. *Brain Science.*

Hui, B.P. et al. (2020, December). Rewards of kindness? A meta-analysis of the link between prosociality and well-being. *Psychological Bulletin.*

Hunt, N. (2013). Memory and social meaning: The impact of society and culture on traumatic memories. In M. Linden & K. Rutkowski (Eds.), *Hurting memories and beneficial forgetting: Posttraumatic stress disorders, biographical developments, and social conflicts* (pp. 49–57). Elsevier.

Johns Hopkins Medicine. (2005). *Healthy diets rich in protein and good fat, and lower in carbs linked to better heart health.*

Kam. J.W. et al. (2021). Distinct electrophysiological signatures of task-unrelated and dynamic thoughts. *Biological Sciences.*

Kok, C.R., et al. (2018, December).Yogurt and other fermented foods as sources of health-promoting bacteria. *Nutrition Review.*

Korb, A. (2012, November).The Grateful Brain. *Psychology Today.*

Kraft, T. (2012, July). Grin and bear it! Smiling facilitates stress recovery. *Association for Psychological Science.*

Li, C. et al. (2017, January). The freedom to pursue happiness: Belief in free will predicts life satisfaction and positive affect among Chinese adolescents. *Frontiers in Psychology.*

Light, K.C., et al. (2005, April). More frequent partner hugs and higher oxytocin levels are linked to lower blood pressure and heart rate in pre-menopausal women. *Biological Psychology,* 69(1), 5-21.

Ocean, N. et al. (2019, February). Lettuce be happy: A longitudinal UK study on the relationship between fruit and vegetable consumption and well-being. *Social Science & Medicine, 222,* 335-345.

Perelman School of Medicine. (2016, November). *Yogic breathing helps fight major depression.*

Phillip, B.A., et al. (2016, July). Increased functional connectivity between cortical hand area and praxis network associated with training-related movements in non-dominant hand precision drawing. *Neuropsychologia,* 1(87), 157-168.

Stellar, J.E. et al. (2015). Positive affect and markers of inflammation: Discrete positive emotions predict lower levels of inflammatory cytokines. *Emotion,* 15(2), 129-133.

University of Gothenburg. (2013, October). People mean most for our collective happiness. *Science Daily.*

University of Virginia Health System. (2017). Probiotic found in yogurt can reverse depression symptoms. *Science Daily.*

Vernon, L. et al. (2009, January). Proactive coping, gratitude, and posttraumatic stress disorder in college women. *Anxiety, Stress, & Coping,* 22(1), 117-127.

Zhao, M. et al. (2022, July). Is free will belief a positive predictor of well-being? The evidence of a cross-lagged examination. *Personality and Individual Differences.*

About the Author

Dr. Lucas holds a Ph.D. in Research Psychology as well as a degree in Chinese Medicine. She has more than 20 years of teaching and speaking experience and is described as "a dynamic speaker who keeps her classes engaged and who can explain complex information in an understandable way." Dr. Lucas believes that Chinese medicine will only thrive in the U.S. if practitioners have the proper skills to offer effective treatment, especially with regard to adequate and correct diagnosis.

Her private practice is based in Denver, Colorado where she specializes in internal medicine. She also sees patients at Littleton Internal Medicine Associates in Littleton Colorado, a perfect setting for modern and Chinese medicine to work together. Her books include *Pulse Diagnosis: Beyond Slippery and Wiry*, *Cosmetic Acupuncture Works!*, the *Mei Zen Cosmetic Acupuncture workbook*, one of her memoirs: *Catholic Daughters of Catholic Mothers: A Memoir and Guided Journal*, and *You don't need Botox* (out of print). She also collaborated with one of her grandchildren on *The Skeleton in a Tutu gets Acupuncture*, and has written countless published articles.

www.acupuncturewoman.com

About the Publisher

ArmLin House is a publisher and production company. We publish your media or help you do it yourself. We can produce your sellable media or create your marketing images and videos. With over thirty years of experience, our team can write, design, and handle the technical details to bring your product to market.

ArmLin House, Inc.
P.O. Box 2522
Littleton, Colorado 80161-2522
contact@armlinhouse.com
www.armlinhouse.com

www.ingramcontent.com/pod-product-compliance
Lightning Source LLC
Chambersburg PA
CBHW060255030426
42335CB00014B/1701